FASTING; YOUR MAIN STRATEGY AGAINST CANCER CELLS

Hidden Secrete To Living A Cancer Free Life

By Julius Abdul

Disclaimer

This book is not intended to replace your medical care, it is not a 100% guaranteed claim that the information contained is going to prevent or cure your cancer.

The information contained in this book is purely researched based on the topic's impact on cancer patients and testimonials evidence of its effect on cancer cell disease from various individuals on the platforms of the likes of Dr. Eric Berge DC and others.

Table Of Content

Introduction

Approximately one in every three Americans will get a kind of cancer during his or her lifetime. One in two men and women will receive a diagnosis at some time in their life according to a claim made in a British statistic publication. Despite these sobering numbers, doctors have made significant progress in understanding the biology of cancer cells, and they have already improved cancer detection and treatment.

Instead of simply waiting for new devices, you can safeguard yourself right now.

Screening tests can help detect cancer in its early stages, but you should always be on the lookout for indications of the disease.

Fasting is without a doubt your best course of action for cancer.

All of these will be covered in this book. The diet for preventing cancer should be different from the diet you would be on if you developed cancer.

This book will reveal all the intricate mechanics of why fasting may be so beneficial to you. It will also outline a different tactic that, if fasting is not an option, can be very helpful.

As you go on, the book will suggest what would be the greatest option if, for instance, a person is too feeble or skinny and needs an alternative to fasting.

One of the earliest treatments still used today is fasting. Long ago, Hippocrates discussed the enormous advantages of fasting. Fasting has historically been a practice of almost every single religion.

Cancer Cells

Understanding some of the differences between healthy cells and malignant cells is crucial. Normal cells can develop into cancerous cells if a certain component of the cell, known as the mitochondria, is damaged. The body's whole energy is produced by the mitochondria, the energy component of every cell. When the mitochondria are injured, the body begins to change its metabolism to a different method of fuel combustion as a means of adaptive survival.

It begins to ferment sugar, at which point it transforms into a cancer cell. After these processes have been completed, the cancer cells will develop a severe glucose need. It also consumes other foods, which will be covered as you read on. However, a cancer cell gets its most fuel from sugar.

Normal cells have a maximum lifespan in the body, after which new ones are generated to replace the dead cells, whereas cancer cells survive forever. This is because normal cells truly have a mortality limit they can live to in the body. Cancer cells take over the body because they multiply more quickly than healthy cells do.

Mechanisms Of Fasting For Cancer
Mechanism 1

The first way that fasting affects a cancer cell is that it helps deprive the cell of its source of energy, specifically glucose, because you're not eating anything and hence not consuming any. By doing this, you help prevent feeding the cancer cell.

Professor Otto Warburg, who received the medical Nobel Prize, made this discovery. Normal cells have a survival edge over cancer cells because they can temporarily ferment sugar under extreme circumstances. Examples include a severe illness like *sepsis (a life-threatening complication of an infection),* a serious *pathogen (an organism causing the disease to its host)* invasion in your body, intensive exercise, or trauma.

Mechanism 2

An amino acid called glutamine and an additional amino acid called arginine can both be used by some malignancies to survive; the issue is that glutamine, which is a component of many proteins, is relatively common. Since it may be found in many different foods, when you fast you won't be consuming glutamine, depriving the cell of this additional fuel.

There are already treatments available that use drugs to restrict glutamine, one of which is "DON," a glutamine inhibitor. Additionally, there are organic glutamine inhibitors and green tea's phytonutrient EGCG. In addition, this has the power to inhibit glutamine, which has an anti-cancer effect. Other phytonutrients included in green tea have a strong anti-cancer effect.

I would want to clarify a few things regarding the glutamine amino acid. If you don't already have cancer, you shouldn't avoid glutamine because doing so won't stop the disease from developing. Glutamate should only be avoided if you have cancer. I must make that clarification for your benefit.

You can't go without eating forever, so what kind of diet will minimize your intake of glutamine and arginine since they are present in so many different meals? Well, if you have cancer, you should avoid a high-protein diet and instead go for a low-protein one. If you're only trying to prevent cancer, I advise sticking to a moderate protein diet because *whey protein* contains a lot of *arginine (a basic amino acid that is a constituent of most proteins).* As a result, I advise staying away from any protein powders, especially whey protein and nuts. Except for the pistachio, which may even have more pistachios on that protocol, these are strong in arginine. These are all related to the protein component.

Mechanism 3

I would like to discuss the idea of autophagy in this third process concerning fasting. Autophagy is a condition rather than a thing; the word "autophagy" means "self-eating," which sounds destructive, but is a very positive survival mechanism in which your body consumes damaged proteins and recycles them into new proteins as well as fuel, making autophagy an alternative fuel source.

Additionally, it can break down waste materials, recycle damaged proteins that aren't being used in any way, fix things, and clean them up. It also has a potent impact on cancer, aids in tumor reduction, and may even prevent the growth of cancer.

Autophagy can take many distinct forms, mitophagy being one of them. What is mitophagy? It refers to the mitochondria's autophagy. Remember how we said that damaged mitochondria are the source of cancer? Well, when you fast, you enhance mitophagy, and your body goes in and starts to clean up the damaged mitochondria.

In addition, autophagy is a very effective anti-inflammatory process, so you'll reduce inflammation, which is important because cancer often spreads into inflammation. It is crucial to keep inflammation at a minimum since people frequently develop cancer in sites of past damage and inflammation.

You'll find it interesting to learn that autophagy also eliminates carcinogens. In the same way, as pesticides, insecticides, herbicides, and fungicides can cause cancer, carcinogens are substances that encourage the development of the disease. Cancer can also be brought on by radiation, however, autophagy cannot remove radiation.

The fact that some circumstances can impair your ability to carry out autophagy is another aspect of this that is crucial. These disorders include obesity, excessive alcohol use, diabetes, viral infections, fatty livers, and chronic inflammation. Because there is less autophagy, all of these chronic factors will raise your risk of developing cancer. If you hadn't guessed, fasting is the primary inducer of autophagy.

Mechanism 4

Your immune system will be the subject of our next mechanism. You must be aware of what fasting can do to your immune system because the two main treatments for cancer are chemotherapy and radiation therapy. Your immune system is a crucial element in both avoiding cancer and directly treating it because both of these things weaken it.

Your immune system has several direct and indirect cancer-killing strategies. Cancer cells can be directly killed by the killer T-cells. The great thing about fasting is that it activates immune system stem cells in your bone marrow to improve your immune system and even repair a damaged immune system. Helper T-cells can indirectly recruit some white blood cells to destroy cancer. Fasting can be included in radiation therapy and chemotherapy routine to lessen the negative effects of radiation and chemotherapy and to increase the efficiency of both treatments.

Since the laws are written so that medical doctors must practice medicine and must adhere to certain protocols to do so, they cannot recommend fasting in place of these other therapies that have side effects without risking losing their license or going to jail. As a result, fasting is never used as the primary treatment but rather as a supplement to medications.

Mechanism 5

Three hormones are the subject of the fifth mechanism, which we will briefly discuss. The liver produces the first one, which is known as IGF-1. Anabolic in nature, this hormone causes things to grow, including muscles. It can also promote the growth of cancer, but I must stress one crucial point: if you don't already have cancer, it won't cause you to develop it. Instead, IGF-1 only promotes the spread of cancer when you already have it, which is why fasting reduces it.

Insulin is the following hormone; like other anabolic hormones, it is known to raise the chance of developing cancer. Since the benefits of fasting are greatly diminished in the presence of insulin and cannot be achieved without lowering insulin levels, maintaining insulin levels low is crucial for maximizing the benefits of fasting and autophagy.

The third one is estrogen, which can cause ovarian, uterine, and breast cancer if it is present in excess. If you're seeking to cure or prevent cancer, you should minimize anything that can raise estrogen because several chemotherapies block the production of estrogen. If you have cancer, you should minimize dairy items like milk. Soy products, particularly soy protein isolates, are also very estrogenic. Birth control pills and hormone replacement therapy also include estrogen, so it's probably not a good idea to take these while you have cancer.

Your estrogen levels can be balanced naturally with iodine from sea kelp. It's excellent for conditions like fibrocystic breast or ovarian cysts, and "Dim" is a concentrated cruciferous product that aids in lowering the amount of estrogen in your body and fights cancer because it comes from cruciferous plants, which is one of the processes utilized to do so.

Mechanism 6

Inflammation is the sixth mechanism, which was briefly addressed before; the more you can reduce inflammation, the lower your risk of developing cancer is. Inflammation is followed by cancer, and many people get cancer from old wounds, including inflamed ones. Dr. Eric Berg DC claims that while he was in practice, a woman who had cancer in a particular area of her breast was asked if she had ever suffered an injury to that area. When she gave it some attention, she realized that shortly after experiencing some trauma, another patient with brain stem cancer entered the hospital.

He asked the second patient if he had ever hurt his brain stem, and the patient said no. "But I did fall off of a roof once and I landed on my head," the patient said, and Dr. Eric informed him that would be an injury to his brain stem, but out of all the things that can get rid of inflammation, fasting is at the top of the list and fasting can also boost the antioxidant networks that you already have in your body, thereby minimizing the free radical damage and lessening inflammation

Mechanism 7

Let's talk about the seventh process regarding fasting to get to this other subject, "ketones." You should be aware at this point that cancer may survive on glucose as well as the amino acids glutamine and arginine. In other words, just because someone is on a ketogenic diet and they are low in sugar does not protect them from getting cancer.

Unfortunately, ketones can give cancer the cellular membrane structure that the cancer cell needs.

Fat-derived ketones serve as the starting point for the membranes that surround cancer cells. Dr. Eric Berg DC in a video said, even though ketones themselves have an anti-tumor effect, he was initially unaware of this new information and tried for a while to suppress it. However, it kept coming up, so he finally dug into some of the research to be satisfied that ketones unfortunately can feed cancer with some of the structural parts that it needs. Herein lies the quandary or issue, but I'll talk about the answer. What can we consume if we aren't allowed to eat carbs, a lot of protein isn't recommended, and fat is also off-limits, remember that we cannot fast forever.

Because the majority of research always begins with mice before moving on to human trials, there has been some study and supported research in Europe linked to a non-toxic technique to inhibit ketones. It had highly intriguing information regarding the differences between cancer cells and healthy cells. It was found that there is only really one chemical mechanism by which ketones may feed the membranes of cancer cells, and if that chemical pathway is blocked, you may be able to starve the cancer of any raw materials for its membranes.

What about normal cells—do they only have one door, as the research raised the question? No, they don't, as was discovered in response to that query. The goal is to block this door, this chemical pathway that is allowing these ketones to make membranes for the cancer cells. This door is called "SCOT," which stands for a very long chemical name that I won't mention in order not to bore you at this time, it is simply scot-inhibitors. Membranes from normal cells can also come from fatty acids, not just ketones.

The scot inhibitors are the ones that are showing the most promise, says Dr. Eric, who is conducting a study on mice in Europe with his team to evaluate the drug area as well as using natural remedies that have fewer side effects on cancer patients. So far, the study has been very successful, he says.

Alpha-lipoic acid, garcinia, red algae, black seed oil, and garlic were also employed. However, garlic handles significantly differently and is crucial. It has a salvage mechanism, which I won't bore you with in detail. All of these scot inhibitors collaborate to help starve the tumor of the building blocks for its cellular membranes.

However, this is a program that I would follow if I had cancer. Before I go into the dosages, I just want you to be aware that I'm not claiming that this would cure or prevent any cancer.

Dr. Eric Berg DC has a strong track record, and he has received positive feedback from those who have adopted his tactics by reading his books and watching his videos on YouTube. He also attests that if he had cancer, he would do this.

A suggestion from Dr. Eric Berg DC: I would start with 0.4 grams of alpha lipoic acid and gradually increase that amount over three weeks to 1.8 grams per day; for garcinia, I would start at 1.2 grams and gradually increase to 3 grams for three weeks; for red algae, I would take eight grams per day; for black seed oil, I would take 500 milligrams twice daily; and for garlic, I would take 500 milligrams four times per day, but that would only be the case if I didn't consume garlic in other ways or during meals.

This treatment is intended to close the "scot" pathway's door, denying cancer the opportunity to obtain the raw materials for its membranes.

The ketogenic diet raises ketones, but fasting raises ketones even more than a ketogenic diet, so how can fasting benefit someone with cancer if it's feeding the cancer cell ketones? This is a different question you might be considering. The reason for this is that many other things are happening while you fast in addition to creating an epigenetic effect that is much greater than the effect of simply ingesting ketones. That, it seems, overrides the mechanism via which ketones feed the cancer membrane through scot.

Fasting For Cancer Prevention

Now we can discuss the fasting protocol. There are two different fasting protocols: one is for prevention, and I'll tell you this for free: the best thing you can do right now is to do whatever you can to prevent cancer. If you don't, once you have cancer, a medical professional will give you all this information and instill fear in you, telling you that you should do this and that you better not do that, leaving you and your friends and family in a state of major confusion.

You should, at the very least, be fasting for roughly 16 hours and have an eight-hour window for eating. The ketogenic diet and intermittent fasting are the best ways to prevent cancer since they will stop the damage to the mitochondria when you eat. It is advised that you consume low-carbohydrate foods.

Once more, what would you do if you were diagnosed with cancer? You should frequently fast for at least 18 hours with a 6-hour window for eating, and if you can, I'd advise you to do more like a 20-hour fast with a 4-hour window for eating, or "OMAD," where you eat One Meal a Day.

In addition, I recommend two days of weekly fasting, which should last between four and eight hours each time. Do two days of calorie restriction if you are unable to fast for two days. To me, that sounds much harder because you haven't really gotten used to it and you're just cutting calories, which means that even a small amount of food can make you feel more hungry. However, studies have shown that calorie-restrictive diets can be effective.

When you eat, the primary meal should be cruciferous vegetables in significant quantity. I would advise fasting for at least four days once a month, but I would also advise going up to seven days if possible. There are many different wonderful meals that you can prepare using this basis of cruciferous vegetables, such as broccoli, kale, cabbage, or cauliflower.

Why is cruciferous food advised? It has significant anti-cancer potential and is minimal in protein, fat, and carbohydrates. The term "anti-angiogenic" refers to a feature that aids in depriving the cancer of its blood vessels; without a blood supply, the cancer cells perish.

Cruciferous vegetables also speed up your liver's phase 1 and phase 2 detoxification processes, which reduces carcinogens. The recommended daily intake is 10 cups, thus if you just eat one meal a day ("omad"), it would only be 10 cups.

You should serve a side dish with modest protein, not heavy protein, such as three ounces of protein. I would advise choosing proteins rich in omega-3 fatty acids, such as those found in fatty fish, sardines, and even cod liver. A person with cancer can benefit greatly from omega-3 fatty acids.

Olive oil is one of the healthiest fats you can eat due to its fantastic anti-cancer characteristics, making it one of the best fats overall. Since cod liver oil contains omega-3, it appears that despite being fat, it won't break down into ketones or provide the cancer cell with the raw materials for its membranes. You will have an even stronger impact on cancer if you can include cruciferous sprouts, such as broccoli sprouts, in addition to avoiding cheese, soy, and conventional foods that contain pesticides. Do mostly organically grown things.

What If You Cannot Fast?

Since I am aware that not everyone will be able to eat this way, this is the researched ideal circumstance. We are conducting this research to learn what we can do to improve the benefits of fasting as well as to develop a strategy for blocking this chemical pathway, or "scot," which would be extremely helpful for patients who just cannot fast due to being too thin, too feeble, or simply unable to do it.

However, in my opinion, ideally, if you fast and follow the nutritional protocols mentioned, it would be a very smart strategy. The research previously mentioned was done to find out the findings of what would happen if someone didn't fast and simply complete these nutritional protocols.

The last point I'd want to make is that, while it's sad that chemotherapy and radiation have a very low success rate and effectiveness, I want to stress that preventing cancer is the most crucial thing you can do right now.

FASTING; YOUR MAIN STRATEGY AGAINST CANCER

Conclusion

It's important to understand the differences between normal cells and cancer cells: Cancer cells originate from normal cells and damage to the mitochondria is what starts the process of a normal cell turning into a cancer cell.

Sugar provides the most fuel for a cancer cell, don't forget that normal cells die, but cancer cells can live forever and cancer cells grow faster than normal cells.

The first mechanism for fasting is that it helps stave off the fuel (glucose) to the cancer cell, secondly, certain cancers can live on glutamine and arginine, which are amino acids. When you fast, you deprive the cancer cell of those types of fuel. Thirdly autophagy may help shrink tumors and inhibit cancer development. The biggest thing that triggers autophagy is fasting. Remember that your immune system is a key factor in preventing cancer and killing cancer. Fasting boosts your immune system and can help regrow a damaged immune system.

Fasting decreases certain hormones that may increase the risk of cancer, such as IGF-1 (this hormone is only a problem if you have cancer), Insulin, and Estrogen. Also, decreasing inflammation helps decrease the risk of cancer. Fasting can help reduce inflammation. Not forgetting that Ketones can provide cancer cells with the cellular membrane structure they need. However, we are currently researching different solutions to this dilemma. Essentially, we need something that can block SCOT. Keep in mind, there are a lot of other things going on when you're fasting that override the mechanism of ketones feeding cancer membranes through SCOT.

The promising natural SCOT inhibitors are Alpha-lipoic acid, Garcinia, Red algae, Black seed oil, and Garlic.
The fasting protocol for cancer prevention is at least 16 hours of fasting with an 8-hour eating window, and a low-carb diet, and the fasting protocol for cancer is at least 18 hours of fasting with a 6-hour eating window. 20 hours of fasting with a four-hour eating window or OMAD would be even better. A 48-hour fast once a week, or two days of 500 calories, or once a month, fast for 4 days and gradually increase to 7 days if possible.

When you eat, the main dish should be cruciferous vegetables (10 cups per day). Consume about 3 ounce of protein high in omega-3 fatty acids. Do not forget that olive oil and cod liver oil are good fats to consume. Broccoli sprouts may also be beneficial.

References

Eric, B. (2022). *Your Strategy Against Cancer* [Video]. Youtube. https://www.youtu.be/hlkhGTGOGaY

American Cancer Society. (2022). ACS guidelines for nutrition and physical activity. Retrieved from https://www.cancer.org/healthy/eat-healthy-get-active/acs-guidelines-nutrition-physical-activity-cancer�prevention/guidelines.html

Bernard, W. S., & Christopher, P. W. (2014). World cancer report 2014. World Health Organization.

Brennan, S. F., Woodside, J. V., Lunny, P. M., Cardwell, C. R., & Cantwell, M. M. (2017). Dietary fat and breast cancer mortality: A systematic review and meta-analysis. Critical Reviews in Food Science and Nutrition, 57(10), 1999-2008. DOI: 10.1080/10408398.2012.724481

Carpenter, D. O., & Bushkin-Bedient, S. (2013). Exposure to chemicals and radiation during childhood and risk for cancer later in life. Journal of Adolescent Health, 52(5), S21-S29. DOI: 10.1016/j.jadohealth.2013.01.027

Chan, D. S., Lau, R., Aune, D., Vieira, R., Greenwood, D. C., Kampman, E., & Norat, T. (2011). Red and processed meat and colorectal cancer incidence: Meta-analysis of prospective studies. PloS One, 6(6), e20456. DOI: 10.1371/journal.pone.0020456

Dahl, W. J., & Stewart, M. L. (2015). Position of the Academy of Nutrition and Dietetics: Health implications of dietary fiber. Journal of the Academy of Nutrition and Dietetics, 115(11), 1861-1870. DOI: 10.1016/j.jand.2015.09.003

Gamage, S. M. K., Dissabandara, L., Lam, A. K. Y., & Gopalan, V. (2018). The role of heme iron molecules derived from red and processed meat in the pathogenesis of colorectal carcinoma. Critical Reviews in Oncology/Hematology, 126, 121-128. DOI: 10.1016/j.critrevonc.2018.03.025

Kerr, J., Anderson, C., & Lippman, S. M. (2017). Physical activity, sedentary behavior, diet, and cancer: an update and emerging new evidence. The Lancet Oncology, 18(8), e457-e471. DOI: 10.1016/S1470-2045(17)30411-4

Lee, J., Shin, A., Oh, J. H., & Kim, J. (2017). Colors of vegetables and fruits and the risks of colorectal cancer. World Journal of Gastroenterology, 23(14), 2527-2538. doi: 10.3748/wjg.v23.i14.2527

Mourouti, N., Panagiotakos, D. B., Kotteas, E. A., & Syrigos, K. N. (2017). Optimizing diet and nutrition for cancer survivors: A review. Maturitas, 105, 33-36. doi: 10.1016/j.maturitas.2017.05.012

Romieu, I. (2019). Dietary factors and cancer. In Encyclopedia of Cancer (3rd ed.). DOI: 10.1016/B978-0-12-801238-3.65036-5

Turati, F., Bravi, F., & La Vecchia, C. (2019). Diet, nutrition, and cancer prevention. In Encyclopedia of Food Security and Sustainability. DOI; 10.1016/B978-0-08-100596-5.22042-8

World Health Organization. (n.d.) Cancer prevention. Retrieved from http://www.who.int/cancer/prevention/en/

www.ingramcontent.com/pod-product-compliance
Lightning Source LLC
Chambersburg PA
CBHW061549250726
48657CB00006B/2378